THE ULTIMATE VEGAN COOKBOOK

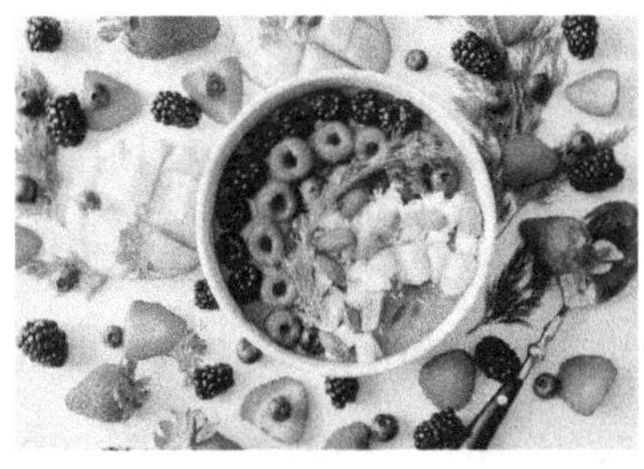

"A Culinary Journcy into the World of Vegan Cuisine"

Britney flowers

TABLE OF CONTENT

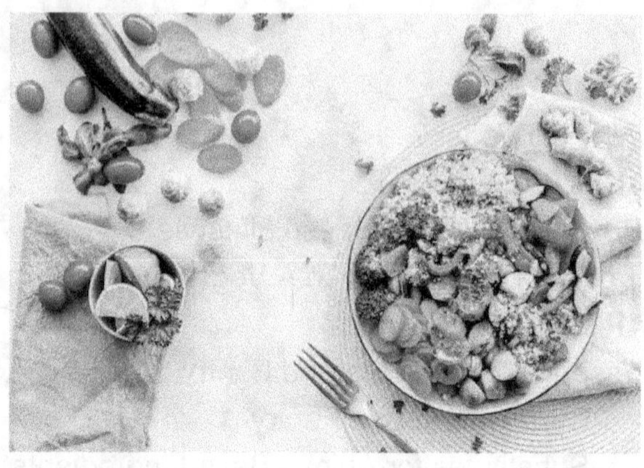

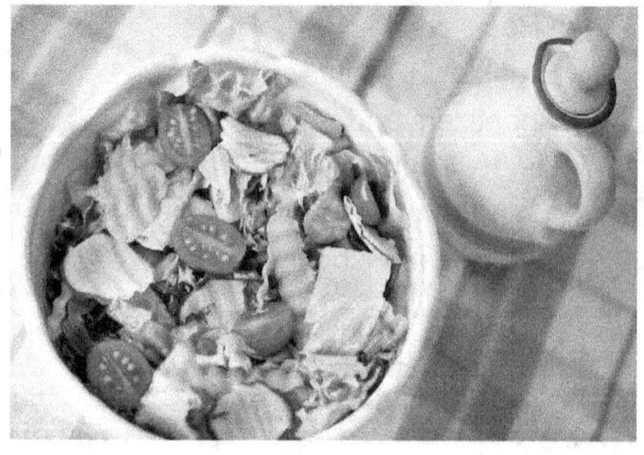

INTRODUCTION

Why Go Vegan?

Welcome to "The Ultimate Vegan Cookbook," a culinary guide that celebrates the vibrant and delicious world of plant-based cuisine. Whether you are a seasoned vegan, curious about adopting a plant-based lifestyle, or simply looking to incorporate more plant-powered meals into your diet, this cookbook is your gateway to a diverse range of mouthwatering and nutritious recipes.

In recent years, veganism has surged in popularity, driven by a growing awareness of its numerous benefits for both our health and the environment. A vegan diet abstains from all animal products, including meat, dairy, eggs, and honey, and instead focuses on consuming plant-based foods such as fruits, vegetables, grains, legumes, nuts, and seeds. By embracing a vegan lifestyle, individuals can reduce their ecological footprint, promote animal welfare, and enhance their own well-being.

"The Vegan Cookbook" is designed to inspire and empower you on your plant-based journey. With its wide array of recipes, it showcases the incredible versatility of plant-based ingredients and dispels the notion that vegan food is bland or restrictive. From delectable breakfasts to hearty main courses, from satisfying soups to indulgent desserts, this cookbook offers a plethora of culinary possibilities that will delight your taste buds and nourish your body.

Whether you are seeking quick and easy meals for busy weekdays, elegant dishes to impress guests, or comforting classics reminiscent of your favorite comfort foods, "The Ultimate Vegan Cookbook" has something for everyone. Each recipe has been thoughtfully crafted to ensure a harmonious blend of flavors, textures, and nutritional balance.

In addition to the recipes themselves, this cookbook also provides valuable information on essential vegan ingredients and pantry staples, guiding you on how to stock your kitchen for success. You will discover alternative options for animal-based ingredients, learn about the benefits of superfoods, and gain a deeper understanding of the building blocks that form the foundation of delicious vegan meals.

Moreover, this book goes beyond the realm of recipes, offering practical advice and cooking tips to enhance your culinary skills. You will learn about knife techniques, cooking methods, and food presentation, enabling you to elevate your creations and unleash your inner chef.

So, whether you are embarking on a lifelong vegan journey or simply looking to incorporate more plant-based meals into your diet, "The Ultimate Vegan Cookbook" is your trusted companion. Get ready to embark on a culinary adventure, where taste, health, and compassion converge on every plate. Let this cookbook be your guide as you explore the endless possibilities of vegan cooking and embrace a lifestyle that nurtures your well-being and honors our planet.

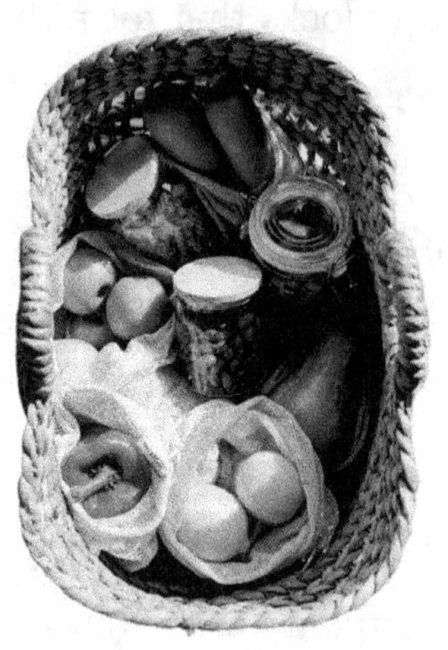

CHAPTER 1

Benefits of a Plant-Based Lifestyle

A plant-based lifestyle offers a wide range of benefits for individuals, animals, and the planet. Here are 15 extensive benefits of adopting a plant-based lifestyle:

1. Improved Heart Health: Plant-based diets are naturally low in saturated fat and cholesterol, reducing the risk of heart disease. They are also rich in heart-healthy nutrients such as fiber, antioxidants, and unsaturated fats, which can lower blood pressure, improve cholesterol levels, and reduce the risk of cardiovascular diseases.

2. Reduced Risk of Chronic Diseases: Plant-based diets have been linked to a decreased risk of chronic diseases such as type 2 diabetes, obesity, certain cancers (such as colorectal, breast, and prostate cancers), and metabolic syndrome. The abundance of plant-based foods provides essential nutrients, antioxidants, and phytochemicals that support overall health and protect against various diseases.

3. Weight Management: Plant-based diets are generally lower in calories and higher in fiber compared to diets that include animal products. This can aid in weight management and contribute to maintaining a healthy body weight. The high fiber content of plant-based foods promotes satiety, reducing overeating and helping to control appetite.

4. Enhanced Digestive Health: The fiber-rich nature of plant-based diets supports a healthy digestive system. Adequate fiber intake

promotes regular bowel movements, prevents constipation, and supports a diverse and thriving gut microbiota. Plant-based foods provide prebiotics, which nourish beneficial gut bacteria and contribute to optimal gut health.

5. Improved Blood Sugar Control: Plant-based diets can help manage blood sugar levels and reduce the risk of developing type 2 diabetes. The fiber, complex carbohydrates, and low glycemic index of plant-based foods contribute to better blood sugar control and insulin sensitivity.

6. Increased Nutritional Intake: A well-planned plant-based lifestyle ensures a diverse and nutrient-rich diet. Plant foods provide essential vitamins (such as vitamin C, vitamin E, folate), minerals (such as potassium, magnesium), and antioxidants. By incorporating a variety of plant-based foods, individuals can meet their nutritional needs and enjoy a well-rounded diet.

7. Reduced Inflammation: Plant-based diets are rich in anti-inflammatory compounds, such as antioxidants and phytochemicals, which can help reduce chronic inflammation in the body. Lowering inflammation levels can alleviate symptoms of inflammatory conditions and reduce the risk of chronic diseases.

8. Enhanced Brain Health: Plant-based diets, particularly those rich in fruits, vegetables, whole grains, and omega-3 fatty acids (found in sources like walnuts and flaxseeds), have been associated with improved cognitive function, memory, and a reduced risk of neurodegenerative diseases like Alzheimer's and dementia.

9. Environmental Sustainability: Choosing a plant-based lifestyle has a positive impact on the environment. Animal agriculture is a significant contributor to greenhouse gas emissions, deforestation, water pollution, and

habitat destruction. By reducing the demand for animal products, individuals can help mitigate climate change, conserve natural resources, and protect biodiversity.

10. Animal Welfare: By adopting a plant-based lifestyle, individuals actively contribute to the welfare and ethical treatment of animals. Avoiding animal products helps reduce the demand for factory farming, which often involves practices that compromise animal welfare. Choosing plant-based alternatives promotes compassion towards animals and supports a more humane food system.

11. Lower Healthcare Costs: Plant-based diets have been associated with lower healthcare costs due to a decreased risk of chronic diseases. By prioritizing preventive health measures through a plant-based lifestyle, individuals can potentially reduce medical expenses related to chronic disease management and medication.

12. Increased Energy and Vitality: Plant-based diets provide abundant nutrients, antioxidants, and phytochemicals that promote increased energy levels and vitality. The high fiber content, coupled with balanced macronutrients, helps stabilize blood sugar levels and sustains energy throughout the day.

13. Improved Skin Health: Plant-based diets, with their abundance of vitamins, minerals, antioxidants, and hydration from plant foods, can contribute to healthier, glowing skin. These diets provide nutrients that support collagen production, promote skin elasticity, and protect against oxidative damage, resulting in improved skin health and a more youthful appearance.

14. Support for Sustainable Food Systems: Embracing a plant-based lifestyle encourages the growth of sustainable food systems. It promotes the cultivation of diverse crops,

reduces reliance on monocultures and intensive farming practices, and fosters local and organic food production. Plant-based diets can help create a more resilient and sustainable food future.

15. Culinary Exploration and Variety: Adopting a plant-based lifestyle opens the door to a world of culinary exploration and creativity. Plant-based diets embrace a wide array of fruits, vegetables, whole grains, legumes, nuts, and seeds, allowing individuals to enjoy a diverse range of flavors, textures, and cuisines. Discovering new plant-based recipes and experimenting with ingredients can make the culinary experience exciting and enjoyable.

Tips for Transitioning To A Vegan Diet

Transitioning to a vegan diet can be an exhilarating and satisfying journey. Below are 20 tips to help you navigate the transition smoothly:

1. Educate Yourself: Learn about the principles and benefits of a vegan diet. Understand the nutritional requirements and familiarize yourself with plant-based sources of essential nutrients like protein, iron, calcium, and vitamin B12.

2. Take it Step by Step: Start by gradually incorporating more plant-based meals into your diet. Begin with a few vegan meals per week and gradually increase the frequency as you become more comfortable and confident.

3. Plan Your Meals: Take time to plan your meals in advance to ensure you have a variety of delicious and nutritious vegan options available. This will help you stay on track and avoid last-minute compromises.

4. Experiment with Recipes: Explore vegan recipes and experiment with new flavors, ingredients, and cooking techniques. There are countless online resources, cookbooks, and apps dedicated to vegan cooking that can inspire your culinary creativity.

5. Find Vegan Alternatives: Discover vegan alternatives for your favorite animal-based foods. There are plant-based alternatives for dairy products, meat substitutes, and even vegan cheeses available in many grocery stores. These can help ease the transition by providing familiar textures and flavors.

6. Focus on Whole Foods: Emphasize whole plant foods such as fruits, vegetables, whole

grains, legumes, nuts, and seeds. These foods are nutrient-dense and provide a wide range of vitamins, minerals, and antioxidants.

7. Stock Your Pantry: Ensure your pantry is well-stocked with vegan staples like grains, legumes, canned beans, nuts, seeds, plant-based milk, herbs, and spices. Having these essentials on hand will make it easier to whip up vegan meals at any time.

8. Embrace Batch Cooking: Prepare larger quantities of meals and store leftovers for future meals. Batch cooking saves time and ensures you always have a healthy vegan meal option available, even on busy days.

9. Connect with the Vegan Community: Join vegan communities online or in your local area. Engaging with like-minded individuals can provide support, encouragement, and a wealth of resources and tips for transitioning to a vegan lifestyle.

10. Read Labels: Develop the habit of reading labels carefully to identify hidden animal-derived ingredients. Be aware of common ingredients such as gelatin, whey, casein, and honey that may be present in processed foods.

11. Be Adventurous with Fruits and Vegetables: Explore a wide variety of fruits and vegetables to diversify your nutrient intake and enjoy new flavors. Try incorporating seasonal produce into your meals for freshness and taste.

12. Substitute Dairy and Eggs: Experiment with plant-based alternatives for dairy and eggs. There are numerous options available, such as almond milk, coconut milk, tofu, tempeh, and chickpea flour, which can replace traditional dairy and egg products in recipes.

13. Seek Support: Share your journey with friends and family, and ask for their support.

Explain your motivations and educate them about the benefits of a vegan lifestyle. Their understanding and encouragement can make the transition easier.

14. Stay Hydrated: Drink plenty of water throughout the day to stay hydrated. Hydration supports total health and helps maintain optimal bodily functions.

15. Learn to Read Menus: When dining out, learn to navigate restaurant menus for vegan options. Many establishments now offer plant-based alternatives or customizable dishes. Don't hesitate to ask for vegan modifications or suggestions from the staff.

16. Be Mindful of Hidden Ingredients: Be aware of hidden animal products in condiments, dressings, sauces, and baked goods. Items like Worcestershire sauce, fish sauce, and honey can be easily overlooked. Opt

for homemade or vegan versions when possible.

17. Find Vegan-Friendly Restaurants: Discover vegan-friendly restaurants in your area. This can make dining out more enjoyable and stress-free. Use online resources, such as restaurant review websites or vegan-specific apps, to find vegan-friendly options near you.

18. Get Creative with Snacks: Find satisfying vegan snack options for when you're on the go. Fresh fruits, raw nuts, hummus and veggie sticks, energy bars, and vegan protein shakes are all convenient and nutritious choices.

19. Be Kind to Yourself: Understand that transitioning to a vegan lifestyle is a personal journey, and everyone's pace is different. Don't be too hard on yourself if you make occasional mistakes or find it challenging initially. Celebrate your growth and concentrate on the positive improvements you are making.

20. Stay Inspired: Stay connected to the vegan community by following vegan influencers, watching documentaries, and reading books about veganism. These resources can provide inspiration, motivation, and a deeper understanding of the positive impact you're making through your choices.

Remember, transitioning to a vegan diet is a process, and it's important to be patient with yourself. Celebrate your successes and enjoy the journey towards a more compassionate and sustainable lifestyle.

CHAPTER 2

Essential Ingredients And Pantry Staples

Building a Vegan Pantry

Building a vegan pantry refers to creating a collection of staple ingredients and pantry items that are suitable for a vegan diet. It involves stocking up on plant-based foods and substitutes to ensure you have a variety of options available for cooking and preparing meals without relying on animal products.

Here are some key components of building a vegan pantry:

1. Grains: Include a variety of whole grains such as quinoa, brown rice, oats, barley, millet, and whole wheat pasta. These serve as a foundation for many vegan meals and provide carbohydrates, fiber, and essential nutrients.

2. Legumes: Stock up on dried legumes like chickpeas, lentils, black beans, kidney beans, and split peas. Legumes are excellent sources of protein, fiber, and minerals and can be used in soups, stews, curries, salads, and even veggie burgers.

3. Nuts and Seeds: Have a selection of nuts and seeds like almonds, walnuts, cashews, chia seeds, flaxseeds, and sunflower seeds. They add texture, flavor, and nutritional value to dishes and can be used in baking, smoothies, sauces, and dressings.

4. Plant-Based Proteins: Consider stocking up on plant-based protein sources like tofu, tempeh, and seitan. These versatile ingredients can be used as meat substitutes in various recipes, offering texture and protein content.

5. Plant-Based Milk: Keep plant-based milk options like almond milk, soy milk, oat milk, or

coconut milk on hand. They can be used in smoothies, cereals, baking, or as a substitute for dairy milk in recipes.

6. Canned Goods: Include canned vegetables, beans, and diced tomatoes in your pantry. These are convenient for quick meals and can be used in recipes like chili, soups, or pasta dishes.

7. Condiments and Sauces: Stock up on vegan condiments and sauces such as soy sauce, tamari, balsamic vinegar, nutritional yeast, tahini, mustard, hot sauce, and plant-based mayonnaise. These add flavor and depth to your dishes.

8. Herbs and Spices: Have a variety of herbs and spices like basil, oregano, thyme, cumin, turmeric, paprika, garlic powder, and onion powder. They enhance the taste of your meals, making them more flavorful and enjoyable.

9. Nutritional Yeast: Nutritional yeast is a popular vegan ingredient that adds a cheesy and nutty flavor to dishes. It can be used as a topping or incorporated into sauces, dressings, or vegan cheese recipes.

10. Baking Essentials: If you enjoy baking, stock up on vegan-friendly baking essentials like flour (all-purpose, whole wheat, or gluten-free), baking powder, baking soda, vegan chocolate chips, and sweeteners like maple syrup or agave nectar.

11. Oils and Fats: Have a selection of cooking oils like olive oil, coconut oil, or avocado oil. Additionally, consider having vegan spreads or margarine for spreading on bread or using in cooking and baking.

12. Specialty Items: Depending on your preferences, consider adding specialty items like vegan mayonnaise, vegan cheese alternatives, tofu-based desserts, plant-based

meat alternatives, or vegan protein powders to your pantry.

By building a vegan pantry, you create a foundation of plant-based ingredients that allow for creativity, variety, and convenience in your vegan cooking and meal preparation. It ensures that you have the necessary ingredients on hand to make satisfying and nutritious vegan meals without relying on animal products.

Substitutes for Animal-Based Ingredients

A vegan diet seeks to exclude all animal-derived products and ingredients, including meat, dairy, eggs, and honey. To create delicious and nutritious meals without using animal-based ingredients, there are numerous vegan substitutes available. Here are some common vegan substitutes for animal-based ingredients:

1. Plant-Based Milk: Replace cow's milk with plant-based alternatives such as almond milk, soy milk, oat milk, coconut milk, or rice milk. These options are readily available and can be used in cooking, baking, or as a dairy milk substitute in beverages and cereals.

2. Tofu: Tofu is a versatile and protein-rich substitute for animal protein. It can be used in stir-fries, curries, scrambles, sandwiches, and even desserts. Tofu comes in different textures, including silken, soft, firm, and extra-firm, providing options for various recipes.

3. Tempeh: Made from fermented soybeans, tempeh is another excellent source of plant-based protein. It has a firm texture and nutty flavor, making it a great substitute for meat in dishes like stir-fries, tacos, sandwiches, and salads.

4. Seitan: Seitan, also known as wheat gluten or wheat meat, is a high-protein substitute for animal-based proteins like beef or chicken. It has a chewy texture and absorbs flavors well, making it suitable for stir-fries, stews, and grilled dishes.

5. Legumes and Beans: Beans and legumes, such as lentils, chickpeas, black beans, and kidney beans, are nutritious and protein-rich ingredients that can replace meat in many dishes. They can be used to make veggie burgers, chili, soups, stews, and pasta sauces.

6. Nutritional Yeast: Nutritional yeast is a deactivated yeast product with a cheesy, nutty flavor. It can be used as a substitute for Parmesan cheese in pasta dishes, sprinkled on popcorn, or incorporated into sauces and dressings.

7. Plant-Based Yogurt: Instead of dairy-based yogurt, opt for plant-based alternatives like soy yogurt, coconut yogurt, or almond milk yogurt. These options can be enjoyed as a standalone snack, added to smoothies, or used in recipes that call for yogurt.

8. Aquafaba: Aquafaba refers to the liquid leftover from cooked chickpeas or canned chickpeas. It can be used as an egg substitute in recipes that require whipping or creating foam, such as meringues, mousses, and mayonnaise.

9.-Based Butter: Replace dairy butter with plant-based alternatives like coconut oil, olive oil, avocado oil, or vegan margarine. These options work well in cooking, baking, and spreading on bread.

10. Vegan Cheese: Several brands offer vegan cheese alternatives made from plant-based ingredients like nuts, soy, or tapioca starch. These cheeses can be used for melting, grating,

or spreading on sandwiches, pizzas, and pasta dishes.

11. Flaxseeds or Chia Seeds: When combined with water, ground flaxseeds or chia seeds create a gel-like consistency that can be used as an egg substitute in baking recipes.

12. Agar Agar or Carrageenan: Agar agar and carrageenan are vegan-friendly alternatives to gelatin. They can be used to create gel-like textures in desserts, jellies, and puddings.

13. Vegetable Broth or Stock: Instead of using meat-based broth or stock, opt for vegetable broth or stock to add flavor to soups, stews, sauces, and risottos.

14. Non-Dairy Ice Cream: Replace traditional dairy ice cream with non-dairy alternatives made from coconut milk, almond milk, or soy milk. These

options come in a variety of flavors and can be enjoyed by vegans and those with lactose intolerance.

15. Vegan Egg Replacers: There are commercially available vegan egg replacers that can be used in baking recipes. These substitutes are specifically formulated to mimic the binding and leavening properties of eggs.

These are just a few examples of the many vegan substitutes available for animal-based ingredients. Experimenting with different options and recipes can lead to exciting and delicious plant-based meals.

CHAPTER 3

Vegan Recipes

• Breakfast Delights

1. Energizing Smoothie Bowls:

Ingredients:

- 2 frozen bananas

- 1 cup frozen berries (such as strawberries, blueberries, or raspberries)

- 1 cup plant-based milk (almond milk, soy milk, or coconut milk)

- Toppings of choice (e.g., sliced fruits, granola, nuts, seeds, coconut flakes)

Instructions:

1. In a blender, combine the frozen bananas, frozen berries, and plant-based milk.

2. Blend until smooth and creamy, adding more milk if needed to reach the desired consistency.

3. Pour the smoothie mixture into a bowl.

4. Top with your favorite toppings, such as sliced fruits, granola, nuts, seeds, and coconut flakes.

5. Enjoy immediately with a spoon.

2. Scrumptious Pancakes and Waffles:

Ingredients:

- 1 ½ cups all-purpose flour (or substitute with whole wheat or gluten-free flour)

- 2 tablespoons sugar (or alternative sweetener of choice)

- 2 teaspoons baking powder

- ½ teaspoon salt

- 1 ¼ cups plant-based milk

- 2 tablespoons vegetable oil (or melted coconut oil)

- 1 teaspoon vanilla extract (optional)

- Additional toppings (e.g., fresh fruits, maple syrup, vegan butter)

Instructions:

1.Whisk the four, salt, baking powder and sugar together in a mixing bowl

2. In a separate bowl, combine the plant-based milk, vegetable oil, and vanilla extract (if using).

3. Pour the wet ingredients into the dry ingredients slowly while turning to barely incorporate. Avoid overmixing; a few lumps are Ok.

4. Preheat a non-stick pan or waffle iron over medium heat.

5. For pancakes: Scoop ¼ cup of batter onto the pan for each pancake then cook until bubbles form on the surface. Flip and cook for another minute or until golden brown.

6. For waffles: Follow the manufacturer's instructions for your waffle iron, greasing it if necessary. Pour the appropriate amount of batter onto the iron and cook until golden brown and crispy.

7. Serve the pancakes or waffles with your favorite toppings, such as fresh fruits, maple syrup, or vegan butter.

3. Creative Oatmeal and Granola Variations:

Ingredients:

- 1 cup rolled oats (gluten-free if needed)
- 2 cups plant-based milk
- Sweetener of choice (such as maple syrup, agave nectar, or dates)
- Optional toppings (e.g., fresh fruits, nuts, seeds, dried fruits, coconut flakes)

Instructions:

1. In a saucepan, combine the rolled oats and plant-based milk.
2. Cook over medium heat, stirring occasionally, until the mixture thickens and the oats are tender. This usually takes about 5-7 minutes.
3. Sweeten the oatmeal to taste with your preferred sweetener. Start with a minimal amount and adjust as desired.
4. Remove the oatmeal from the heat and let it cool slightly.
5. Transfer the oatmeal to serving bowls.

6. Add your favorite toppings, such as fresh fruits, nuts, seeds, dried fruits, or coconut flakes.

7. Alternatively, you can make homemade granola by spreading the cooked oats on a baking sheet and baking at a low temperature (around 300°F or 150°C) until crispy. Add your desired mix-ins like nuts, seeds, and dried fruits before baking.

8. Allow the granola to cool completely before storing it in an airtight container.

9. Serve the oatmeal or granola variations as a nourishing and customizable breakfast option.

• Appetizers and Snacks

1. Flavorful Dips and Spreads:

Ingredients:

- 1 cup cooked chickpeas

- 2 tablespoons tahini

- 2 tablespoons lemon juice

- 2 tablespoons olive oil

- 1 clove garlic, minced

- Salt and pepper to taste

- Optional: herbs, spices, or additional flavorings (e.g., cumin, paprika, roasted red peppers, sun-dried tomatoes)

Instructions:

1. In a food processor or blender, combine the cooked chickpeas, tahini, lemon juice, olive oil, garlic, salt, and pepper.

2. Blend until smooth and creamy, adding a little water if needed to achieve the desired consistency.

3. Taste and adjust the seasonings as desired.

4. If you'd like to add extra flavor, incorporate herbs, spices, or other optional ingredients to customize the dip or spread.

5. Transfer the dip or spread to a serving bowl and refrigerate for at least 30 minutes before serving to allow the flavors to meld.

6. Serve with raw vegetables, pita bread, crackers, or use as a sandwich spread.

2. Mouthwatering Bites and Finger Foods:

Ingredients:

- 1 block of firm tofu, drained and pressed

- 2 tablespoons soy sauce or tamari

- 2 tablespoons maple syrup or agave nectar

- 1 tablespoon sesame oil

- 1 clove garlic, minced

- Optional: additional seasonings or spices (e.g., ginger, chili powder, paprika, herbs)

Instructions:

1. Preheat the oven to 400°F (200°C) and line a baking sheet with parchment paper.

2. Cut the pressed tofu into bite-sized pieces or sticks.

3. In a bowl, whisk together the soy sauce or tamari, maple syrup or agave nectar, sesame oil, garlic, and any optional seasonings.

4. Add the tofu pieces to the marinade and toss gently to coat.

5. Let the tofu marinate for at least 15 minutes, allowing the flavors to infuse.

6. Arrange the tofu pieces on the prepared baking sheet, leaving space between them.

7. Bake in the preheated oven for 20-25 minutes, or until the tofu is golden brown and crispy on the outside.

8. Serve the mouthwatering bites and finger foods as an appetizer or snack, with dipping sauces if desired.

3. Fresh and Crunchy Salads:

Ingredients:

- Mixed salad greens (such as lettuce, spinach, arugula)

- Assorted vegetables (e.g., cherry tomatoes, cucumbers, bell peppers, carrots, radishes, avocados)

- Optional additions: nuts, seeds, dried fruits, croutons, vegan cheese, cooked grains or legumes

- Dressing: olive oil, vinegar (such as balsamic or apple cider vinegar), lemon juice, Dijon mustard, salt, pepper, herbs (e.g., basil, parsley, dill)

Instructions:

1. Wash and prepare the salad greens and vegetables by slicing, dicing, or chopping them into bite-sized pieces.

2. Place the salad greens in a large bowl and add the prepared vegetables.

3. If desired, add additional toppings such as nuts, seeds, dried fruits, croutons, vegan cheese, or cooked grains or legumes.

4. In a small bowl, whisk together the dressing ingredients, adjusting the quantities to taste.

5. Drizzle the dressing over the salad and toss gently to combine, ensuring all ingredients are coated.

6. Serve the fresh and crunchy salad as a side dish or a main course.

• Hearty Soups and Stews

1. Comforting Lentil Soup:

Ingredients:

- 1 cup dried lentils (green or brown), rinsed and drained
- 1 onion, diced
- 2 carrots, diced
- 2 celery stalks, diced
- 3 cloves garlic, minced
- 1 can diced tomatoes
- 4 cups vegetable broth
- 1 teaspoon ground cumin
- 1 teaspoon ground coriander
- 1/2 teaspoon turmeric
- Salt and pepper to taste
- Fresh lemon juice (optional)
- Fresh cilantro or parsley for garnish (optional)

Instructions:

1. In a large pot, heat some oil over medium heat.

2. Add the diced onion, carrots, and celery to the pot and sauté until the vegetables are softened.

3. Add the minced garlic, cumin, coriander, and turmeric to the pot, and stir for about a minute to release their flavors.

4. Add the lentils, diced tomatoes (with their juices), and vegetable broth to the pot. Stir well to combine.

5. Bring the mixture to a boil, then reduce the heat to a simmer. Cover the pot and let it cook for about 25-30 minutes or until the lentils are tender.

6. Season the soup with salt and pepper to taste. If desired, add a squeeze of fresh lemon juice for a touch of brightness.

7. Serve the comforting lentil soup hot, garnished with fresh cilantro or parsley if desired.

2. Creamy Roasted Vegetable Chowder:

Ingredients:

- Assorted vegetables for roasting (e.g., potatoes, carrots, bell peppers, cauliflower, butternut squash)
- 1 onion, diced
- 2 cloves garlic, minced
- 4 cups vegetable broth
- 1 cup plant-based milk (such as almond milk or coconut milk)
- 2 tablespoons flour (gluten-free if needed)
- 1 teaspoon dried thyme
- 1/2 teaspoon smoked paprika
- Salt and pepper to taste
- Fresh herbs for garnish (e.g., parsley, chives)

Instructions:

1. Preheat the oven to 400°F (200°C).

2. Chop the vegetables into bite-sized pieces and spread them on a baking sheet.

3. Drizzle with olive oil and season with salt and pepper. Roast the vegetables in the

preheated oven for about 25-30 minutes or until they are tender and lightly browned.

4. In a large pot, sauté the diced onion and minced garlic until softened.

5. Add the roasted vegetables to the pot, along with the vegetable broth, dried thyme, and smoked paprika. Stir well to combine.

6. In a separate bowl, whisk together the plant-based milk and flour until smooth.

7. Pour the milk-flour mixture into the pot, stirring constantly to prevent lumps from forming.

8. Bring the chowder to a simmer and let it cook for about 15-20 minutes, stirring occasionally, until it thickens and the flavors meld.

9. Season with salt and pepper to taste.

10. Serve the creamy roasted vegetable chowder hot, garnished with fresh herbs.

3. Spicy Chickpea Stew:

Ingredients:

- 2 tablespoons olive oil

- 1 onion, diced

- 3 cloves garlic, minced

- 1 bell pepper, diced

- 2 carrots, diced

- 1 can diced tomatoes

- 2 cups vegetable broth

- 2 teaspoons ground cumin

- 1 teaspoon smoked paprika

- 1/2 teaspoon chili powder (adjust to taste)

- 1 can chickpeas, drained and rinsed

- Salt and pepper to taste

- Fresh cilantro for garnish (optional)

Instructions:

1. Heat the olive oil in a large pot over medium heat.

2. Add the diced onion, minced garlic, bell pepper, and carrots to the pot. Sauté until the vegetables are softened.

3. Add the diced tomatoes (with their juices), vegetable broth, ground cumin, smoked paprika, and chili powder to the pot. Stir well to combine.

4. Bring the mixture to a boil, then reduce the heat to a simmer. Cover the pot and let it cook for about 15-20 minutes to allow the flavors to meld.

5. Add the drained and rinsed chickpeas to the pot and stir to incorporate them.

6. Continue simmering for another 5-10 minutes, until the chickpeas are heated through and the stew has thickened slightly.

7. Season with salt and pepper to taste.

8. Serve the spicy chickpea stew hot, garnished with fresh cilantro if desired.

• **Main Course Marvels**

1. Satisfying Pasta and Grain-Based Dishes:

Ingredients:

- Pasta or grains of choice (e.g., spaghetti, penne, quinoa, rice)

- Assorted vegetables (e.g., bell peppers, zucchini, mushrooms, cherry tomatoes)

- Sauce or dressing of choice (e.g., marinara sauce, pesto, lemon garlic sauce)

- Optional additions: vegan cheese, fresh herbs, nutritional yeast, crushed red pepper flakes

Instructions:

1. Cook the pasta or grains according to the package instructions until al dente. Drain and set aside.

2. Meanwhile, prepare the vegetables by washing and chopping them into bite-sized pieces.

3. In a pan, heat some oil over medium heat and add the vegetables. Stir-fry until they are cooked to your desired tenderness.

4. Add the cooked pasta or grains to the pan with the vegetables and mix well.

5. Pour in the sauce or dressing of your choice and toss until everything is evenly coated.

6. If desired, add any optional additions such as vegan cheese, fresh herbs, nutritional yeast, or crushed red pepper flakes for extra flavor.

7. Cook for an additional minute or two to heat through.

8. Serve the satisfying pasta or grain-based dish hot, garnished with additional toppings if desired.

2. Flavor-Packed Vegetable Stir-Fries:

Ingredients:

- Assorted vegetables (e.g., broccoli, carrots, snap peas, bell peppers, onions)

- Sauce of choice (e.g., soy sauce, teriyaki sauce, peanut sauce)

- Oil for cooking (e.g., sesame oil, olive oil)

-   Optional additions: tofu, tempeh, mushrooms, garlic, ginger, sesame seeds

Instructions:

1. Wash and chop the vegetables into bite-sized pieces.

2. In a large pan or wok, heat some oil over medium-high heat.

3. Add the vegetables to the pan and stir-fry them until they are cooked but still crisp.

4. If using tofu or tempeh, add them to the pan and cook until they are heated through.

5. In a small bowl, whisk together the sauce ingredients.

6. Pour the sauce over the stir-fried vegetables and mix well to coat evenly.

7. If desired, add any optional additions such as mushrooms, garlic, ginger, or sesame seeds to enhance the flavor.

8. Cook for an additional minute or two to allow the flavors to meld.

9. Serve the flavor-packed vegetable stir-fry hot over rice, noodles, or alongside grains.

3. Protein-Rich Tofu and Tempeh Creations:

Ingredients:

- Firm tofu or tempeh, cut into desired shapes (e.g., cubes, strips)
- Marinade or sauce of choice (e.g., soy sauce, barbecue sauce, curry paste)
- Oil for cooking (e.g., canola oil, coconut oil)
- Optional additions: vegetables, herbs, spices, nutritional yeast

Instructions:

1. In a shallow dish, prepare the marinade or sauce by combining the desired ingredients.

2. Add the tofu or tempeh to the dish and coat it evenly with the marinade or sauce. Let it marinate for at least 15 minutes to absorb the flavors.

3. In a skillet or pan, heat some oil over medium-high heat.

4. Add the marinated tofu or tempeh to the pan and cook until it is golden brown and crispy on all sides.

5. If desired, add vegetables, herbs, spices, or nutritional yeast to the pan to enhance the flavor and texture.

6. Continue cooking until the tofu or tempeh is heated through and the additional ingredients are cooked to your preference.

7. Serve the protein-rich tofu or tempeh creations hot, alongside grains, in wraps, or as a protein component in various dishes.

• Oven-Baked Goodness

1. Delicious Veggie Casseroles:

Ingredients:

- Assorted vegetables (e.g., potatoes, carrots, broccoli, cauliflower, bell peppers)

- Sauce or base (e.g., tomato sauce, creamy cashew sauce, vegan cheese sauce)

- Herbs and spices (e.g., garlic powder, onion powder, dried thyme, dried basil)

- Optional additions: cooked grains, vegan protein (e.g., lentils, chickpeas), breadcrumbs

Instructions:

1. Preheat the oven to 375°F (190°C).

2. Wash and chop the vegetables into bite-sized pieces.

3. In a baking dish, layer the vegetables evenly.

4. In a separate bowl, mix together the sauce or base with your choice of herbs and spices.

5. Pour the sauce or base mixture over the vegetables, ensuring they are well coated.

6. If desired, add any optional additions such as cooked grains or vegan protein to the casserole.

7. Cover the baking dish with foil and bake in the preheated oven for about 30-40 minutes, or until the vegetables are tender.

8. Remove the foil and sprinkle breadcrumbs over the top, if desired.

9. Return the casserole to the oven and bake for an additional 10 minutes, or until the top is golden and crispy.

10. Serve the delicious veggie casserole hot as a main dish or a side.

2. Tasty Stuffed Peppers and Squashes:

Ingredients:

- Bell peppers or squashes of choice (e.g., bell peppers, zucchini, acorn squash, butternut squash)

- Stuffing ingredients (e.g., cooked grains, diced vegetables, beans, vegan cheese)

- Sauce or seasoning (e.g., marinara sauce, soy sauce, herbs and spices)

- Optional additions: breadcrumbs, vegan parmesan cheese

Instructions:

1. Preheat the oven to 375°F (190°C).

2. Cut the tops off the bell peppers or squashes and remove the seeds and membranes.

3. In a bowl, mix together the stuffing ingredients of your choice. Be creative and combine different flavors and textures.

4. Stuff the bell peppers or squashes with the mixture, packing it tightly.

5. Place the stuffed bell peppers or squashes in a baking dish.

6. Drizzle the sauce or sprinkle the desired seasoning over the top of the stuffed vegetables.

7. If desired, sprinkle breadcrumbs and vegan parmesan cheese over the top for added texture and flavor.

8. Cover the baking dish with foil and bake in the preheated oven for about 30-40 minutes, or until the bell peppers or squashes are tender.

9. Remove the foil and bake for an additional 10 minutes, or until the top is golden and crispy.

10. Serve the tasty stuffed peppers and squashes hot as a satisfying and flavorful meal.

3. Savory Baked Tofu and Seitan:

Ingredients:

- Firm tofu or seitan, cut into desired shapes (e.g., cubes, slices)

- Marinade or seasoning (e.g., soy sauce, barbecue sauce, garlic and herb marinade)

- Oil for greasing the baking dish

- Optional additions: vegetables, herbs, spices

Instructions:

1. Preheat the oven to 375°F (190°C).

2. In a shallow dish, prepare the marinade or seasoning by combining the desired ingredients.

3. Add the tofu or seitan to the dish and coat it evenly with the marinade or seasoning. Let it marinate for at least 15 minutes to absorb the flavors.

4. Grease a baking dish with oil to prevent sticking.

5. Arrange the marinated tofu or seitan in a single layer in the baking dish.

6. If desired, add vegetables, herbs, or spices to the dish for additional flavor.

7. Bake in the preheated oven for about 20-25 minutes, flipping halfway through, or until the tofu or seitan is browned and crispy on the outside.

8. Remove from the oven and let it cool slightly before serving.

9. Serve the savory baked tofu or seitan hot as a protein-rich centerpiece or as a flavorful addition to various dishes.

• Sensational Sauces and Dressings

1. Homemade Vegan Cheese Sauces:

Ingredients:

- Cashews or almonds, soaked overnight and drained

- Nutritional yeast

- Plant-based milk (e.g., almond milk, soy milk)

- Lemon juice or apple cider vinegar

- Garlic powder

- Onion powder

- Salt and pepper to taste

- Optional additions: smoked paprika, turmeric, miso paste, Dijon mustard

Instructions:

1. In a blender or food processor, combine the soaked cashews or almonds, nutritional yeast, plant-based milk, lemon juice or apple cider vinegar, garlic powder, onion powder, salt, and pepper.

2. Blend until smooth and creamy. If needed, add more plant-based milk to achieve the desired consistency.

3. Taste the sauce and adjust the seasonings according to your preference.

4. For different variations, add optional additions such as smoked paprika for a smoky flavor, turmeric for a vibrant yellow color, miso paste for umami notes, or Dijon mustard for tanginess.

5. Blend again to incorporate any additional ingredients.

6. Transfer the homemade vegan cheese sauce to a saucepan and heat over low heat, stirring continuously, until warmed through.

7. Use the vegan cheese sauce as a delicious topping for nachos, pasta, pizza, or as a dip for vegetables.

2. Zesty Salad Dressings:

Ingredients:

- Olive oil or other plant-based oil

- Vinegar (e.g., balsamic vinegar, apple cider vinegar)

- Lemon juice

- Dijon mustard

- Maple syrup or agave nectar

- Garlic clove, minced

- Salt and pepper to taste

- Optional additions: herbs (e.g., basil, cilantro), spices (e.g., paprika, cayenne pepper), tahini

Instructions:

1. In a small bowl, whisk together the olive oil, vinegar, lemon juice, Dijon mustard, maple syrup or agave nectar, minced garlic, salt, and pepper.

2. Taste the dressing and adjust the ingredients according to your preference.

3. For different flavor profiles, add optional additions such as herbs (e.g., basil, cilantro) for freshness, spices (e.g., paprika, cayenne pepper) for a kick, or tahini for creaminess.

4. Whisk again to incorporate any additional ingredients.

5. Transfer the zesty salad dressing to a jar or container and refrigerate for at least 30 minutes to allow the flavors to meld.

6. Shake the dressing well before using it on your favorite salads.

3. Flavor-Enhancing Condiments:

Ingredients:

- Vegan mayonnaise

- Mustard (e.g., Dijon mustard, whole grain mustard)

- Ketchup (look for vegan-friendly options)

- Sriracha or hot sauce

- Soy sauce or tamari (gluten-free option)

- Worcestershire sauce (look for vegan-friendly options)

- Pickles or pickle relish

- Lemon juice

- Optional additions: minced garlic, chopped herbs (e.g., parsley, chives), nutritional yeast, liquid smoke

Instructions:

1. In separate small bowls, prepare each condiment by combining the ingredients according to the desired flavor.

2. For vegan mayonnaise-based condiments, mix vegan mayonnaise with different ingredients such as mustard, minced garlic,

chopped herbs, nutritional yeast, or lemon juice to create variations.

3. Adjust the quantities of each ingredient to achieve the desired taste.

4. For a tangy and spicy condiment, mix together ketchup, sriracha or hot sauce, soy sauce or tamari, and a squeeze of lemon juice.

5. For a smoky and savory condiment, combine Worcestershire sauce, liquid smoke, soy sauce or tamari, and minced garlic.

6. Stir each condiment well to ensure all the ingredients are evenly incorporated.

7. Transfer the flavor-enhancing condiments to jars or containers and refrigerate until ready to use.

8. Use these condiments to add extra flavor to burgers, sandwiches, wraps, or as dipping sauces for fries or snacks.

• **Decadent Desserts**

1. Indulgent Chocolate Treats:

Ingredients:

- Vegan chocolate (dark, semi-sweet, or milk chocolate depending on preference)
- Coconut oil or vegan butter
- Sweetener of choice (e.g., maple syrup, agave nectar, coconut sugar)
- Optional additions: nuts, dried fruits, shredded coconut, sea salt, vanilla extract

Instructions:

1. Melt the vegan chocolate in a microwave-safe bowl or over a double boiler.

2. Stir in coconut oil or vegan butter and sweetener of choice until well combined.

3. If desired, add optional additions such as nuts, dried fruits, shredded coconut, a pinch of sea salt, or a splash of vanilla extract for added flavor and texture.

4. Pour the mixture into molds or spread it evenly onto a parchment-lined baking sheet.

5. Place the molds or baking sheet in the refrigerator or freezer until the chocolate is set.

6. Once set, remove from the molds or break into desired pieces.

7. Store the indulgent chocolate treats in an airtight container in the refrigerator to maintain freshness.

2. Fruit-Based Delicacies:

Ingredients:

- Assorted fruits (e.g., berries, bananas, mangoes, peaches)
- Coconut cream or non-dairy yogurt
- Sweetener of choice (e.g., maple syrup, agave nectar, dates)
- Optional additions: nuts, seeds, granola, shredded coconut, cocoa powder

Instructions:

1. Wash and prepare the fruits by peeling, slicing, or dicing them as desired.

2. In a bowl, combine the coconut cream or non-dairy yogurt with the sweetener of choice, adjusting the sweetness to your preference.

3. If desired, add optional additions such as nuts, seeds, granola, shredded coconut, or a sprinkle of cocoa powder for added texture and flavor.

4. Layer the fruit and coconut cream or non-dairy yogurt mixture in serving glasses or bowls.

5. Repeat the layers until all the ingredients are used, finishing with a dollop of the coconut cream or non-dairy yogurt on top.

6. Refrigerate the fruit-based delicacies for at least 30 minutes to allow the flavors to meld.

7. Serve the fruit-based delicacies chilled as a refreshing and nutritious dessert.

3. Creamy Vegan Cheesecakes and Pies:

Ingredients:

- Vegan cream cheese or cashews (soaked overnight and drained)

- Coconut cream or non-dairy yogurt

- Sweetener of choice (e.g., maple syrup, agave nectar, coconut sugar)
- Crust ingredients (e.g., crushed cookies, nuts, dates)
- Optional additions: fruit compote, chocolate ganache, crushed nuts for topping

Instructions:

1. Prepare the crust by combining the crust ingredients in a food processor until they form a sticky mixture.

2. Press the crust mixture into the bottom of a springform pan or individual pie tins, creating an even layer.

3. In a blender or food processor, combine the vegan cream cheese or soaked cashews, coconut cream or non-dairy yogurt, and sweetener of choice. Blend until smooth and creamy.

4. If desired, add optional additions such as fruit compote, chocolate ganache, or crushed nuts to the cream cheese or cashew mixture for added flavor and texture.

5. Pour the cream cheese or cashew mixture onto the crust in the springform pan or individual pie tins, smoothing the top with a spatula.

6. Place the cheesecake or pie in the refrigerator for at least 4-6 hours, or until it is set.

7. Once set, remove from the pan or tins and garnish with additional toppings if desired.

8. Slice and serve the creamy vegan cheesecakes and pies chilled as a delectable and indulgent dessert.

Beverages and Refreshments

1. Nutritious Smoothies and Juices:

Ingredients:

- Assorted fruits (e.g., bananas, berries, mangoes, pineapple)

- Leafy greens (e.g., spinach, kale)

- Plant-based milk or water

- Optional additions: nut butter, chia seeds, flaxseeds, protein powder, sweetener of choice (e.g., maple syrup, agave nectar)

Instructions:

1. Choose your desired combination of fruits and leafy greens. Wash and prepare them by peeling, slicing, or removing any stems or pits.

2. In a blender, combine the fruits, leafy greens, and plant-based milk or water.

3. Add optional additions such as nut butter, chia seeds, flaxseeds, protein powder, or a sweetener of choice for added nutrition and flavor.

4. Blend the ingredients until smooth and creamy, adjusting the consistency by adding more liquid if needed.

5. Taste the smoothie or juice and adjust the sweetness or flavors according to your preference.

6. Pour the nutritious smoothie or juice into a glass or jar, and serve immediately for maximum freshness and nutrients.

2. Energizing Coffee and Tea Blends:

Ingredients:

- Coffee beans or ground coffee (for coffee blends)

- Assorted tea leaves or tea bags (for tea blends)

- Plant-based milk or creamer

- Optional additions: sweetener of choice (e.g., maple syrup, agave nectar), spices (e.g., cinnamon, nutmeg), flavor extracts (e.g., vanilla extract, almond extract)

Instructions:

1. Brew a fresh pot of coffee using your preferred method or prepare a cup of tea with hot water and the desired tea leaves or tea bags.

2. While the coffee or tea is brewing, heat plant-based milk or creamer in a saucepan or microwave until warm.

3. If desired, add optional additions such as sweetener of choice, spices, or flavor extracts to

the warmed plant-based milk or creamer, stirring until well combined.

4. Pour the brewed coffee or tea into a mug, leaving room for the plant-based milk or creamer.

5. Slowly pour the warmed plant-based milk or creamer into the coffee or tea, stirring gently to incorporate.

6. Taste the energizing coffee or tea blend and adjust the sweetness or flavors as desired.

7. Garnish with a sprinkle of spices or a drizzle of sweetener, if desired.

8. Enjoy the energizing coffee or tea blend hot for a comforting and invigorating beverage.

3. Creative Mocktails and Refreshing Drinks:

Ingredients:

- Assorted fruit juices (e.g., orange juice, pineapple juice, cranberry juice)
- Sparkling water or soda water
- Citrus fruits (e.g., lemons, limes)
- Fresh herbs (e.g., mint, basil)

- Optional additions: agave syrup, flavored syrups, fruit slices for garnish

Instructions:

1. In a pitcher or individual glasses, combine the assorted fruit juices with sparkling water or soda water. Adjust the ratios based on your taste preferences.

2. Squeeze fresh citrus fruits, such as lemons or limes, into the mixture for a tangy twist.

3. Tear or lightly crush fresh herbs like mint or basil and add them to the pitcher or glasses for a refreshing aroma and flavor.

4. If desired, add optional additions such as agave syrup or flavored syrups to enhance the sweetness or add different flavors.

5. Stir gently to mix the ingredients together.

6. Fill serving glasses with ice cubes and pour the creative mocktails or refreshing drinks over the ice.

7. Garnish the drinks with fruit slices or herb sprigs for an appealing presentation.

8. Serve the creative mocktails and refreshing drinks immediately to enjoy their vibrant flavors and coolness.

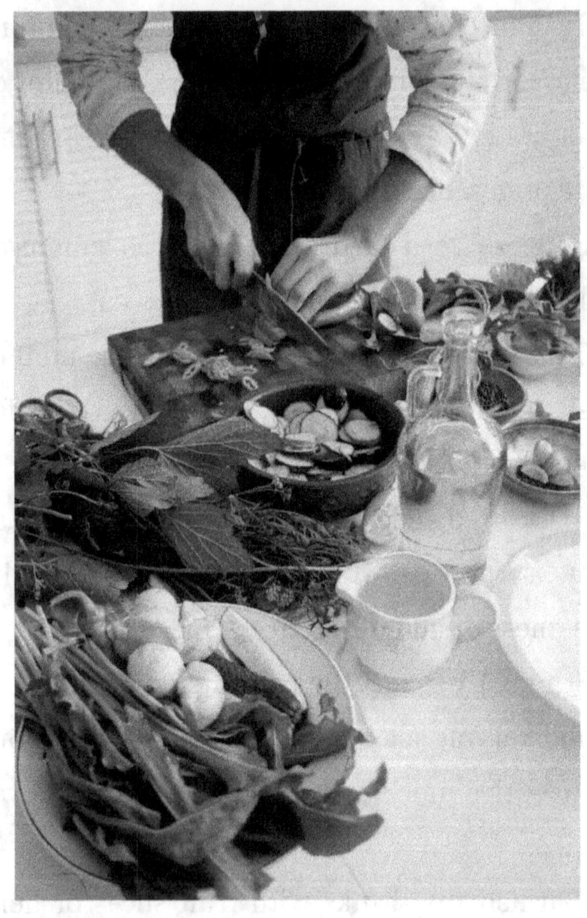

CHAPTER 4

Vegan Cooking Tips and Techniques

Knife Skills And Cooking Methods

Knife Skills for a Vegan Diet:

1. Grip and Handling: Hold the knife with a firm grip, ensuring your fingers are curled under and your thumb is placed on the side of the blade. This provides control and reduces the risk of accidents.

2. Chopping: To chop vegetables or fruits, start by cutting them into manageable pieces. Hold the item securely and use a rocking motion to guide the knife through the ingredients, keeping the tip of the knife on the cutting board.

3. Dicing: Dicing involves cutting ingredients into small, uniform cubes. Start by slicing the vegetable into even planks, then stack the planks and cut them into strips. Finally, chop the strips into cubes.

4. Mincing: Mincing refers to finely chopping ingredients. Begin by finely slicing the item, then gather the slices together and chop them into smaller pieces. Continue chopping until you achieve the desired fineness.

5. Julienne: Julienne is a technique used to create long, thin strips of vegetables. Start by cutting the ingredient into rectangular planks, then stack the planks and cut them into matchstick-like strips.

6. Slicing: Slicing involves cutting ingredients into thin, even pieces. Place the item on the cutting board and use a steady back-and-forth motion with the knife to create thin slices.

Cooking Methods for a Vegan Diet:

1. Sautéing: Heat a small amount of oil or vegetable broth in a pan and cook the ingredients over medium heat, stirring frequently. This method works well for quickly cooking vegetables, tofu, or tempeh.

2. Stir-Frying: Similar to sautéing, stir-frying involves cooking ingredients over high heat in a pan or wok. Use a small amount of oil and continuously stir the ingredients to evenly cook them.

3. Steaming: Steaming involves cooking ingredients using steam. Place the ingredients in a steamer basket or a colander over boiling water and cover with a lid. This method is ideal for vegetables, grains, and dumplings.

4. Roasting/Baking: Roasting or baking involves cooking ingredients in the oven at high heat. Arrange the ingredients on a baking sheet and drizzle them with oil or marinade. This

method is great for root vegetables, tofu, or cauliflower steaks.

5. Boiling: Boiling is a common method for cooking grains, legumes, and pasta. Place the ingredients in a pot with enough water to cover them, and cook until tender.

6. Grilling: Grilling imparts a smoky flavor to ingredients. Place vegetables, tofu, or tempeh on a grill or grill pan, and cook over medium-high heat, flipping them occasionally until charred and tender.

By mastering these knife skills and cooking methods, you'll have the foundation to create a wide range of delicious vegan meals. Remember to practice proper knife handling and explore different cooking techniques to enhance your culinary skills.

Food Presentation And Garnishing

Food presentation and garnishing play an essential role in enhancing the visual appeal of a dish and making it more enticing. Here are some key points to consider for food presentation and garnishing in a vegan diet:

1. Plate Selection: Choose plates or bowls that complement the colors and textures of the dish. Consider using white or neutral-colored plates to let the vibrant colors of the vegan ingredients stand out.

2. Balance and Composition: Create a balanced and visually appealing arrangement of the different components of the dish. Use the principles of symmetry, asymmetry, and

negative space to create an attractive composition.

3. Colorful Ingredients: Use a variety of colorful fruits, vegetables, and herbs to add visual interest to the dish. Vibrant greens, reds, oranges, and purples can create a visually stunning plate.

4. Layering and Stacking: Utilize layering and stacking techniques to create height and depth in your presentation. Stack ingredients like grilled vegetables or tofu, or layer different components of a dish for an appealing visual effect.

5. Garnishing with Herbs and Greens: Sprinkle fresh herbs, such as basil, parsley, or cilantro, over the dish to add a pop of color and freshness. Edible flowers or microgreens can also be used to garnish salads, soups, or appetizers.

6. Sauces and Drizzles: Use vegan sauces, such as pesto, tahini, or cashew cream, to add artistic swirls or drizzles on the plate. These sauces not only enhance the flavor but also add visual appeal to the dish.

7. Texture and Crunch: Incorporate crispy elements like toasted nuts, seeds, or croutons to provide texture contrast to the dish. Sprinkle them on top or place them strategically for added visual interest.

8. Utensil Placement: Consider the placement of utensils, such as forks, spoons, or chopsticks, when presenting your dish. They can be arranged neatly beside or on top of the plate, or rolled in a napkin for a more formal presentation.

9. Negative Space: Allow for some empty space on the plate to create a clean and visually pleasing presentation. This negative space

helps the main ingredients stand out and adds a sense of elegance to the dish.

10. Attention to Detail: Pay attention to the small details, such as wiping off any excess sauce or arranging ingredients neatly. These details contribute to a polished and professional presentation.

Remember, food presentation is a creative process, so feel free to experiment and develop your own unique style. By considering these tips, you can create visually stunning and appetizing vegan dishes that are sure to impress.

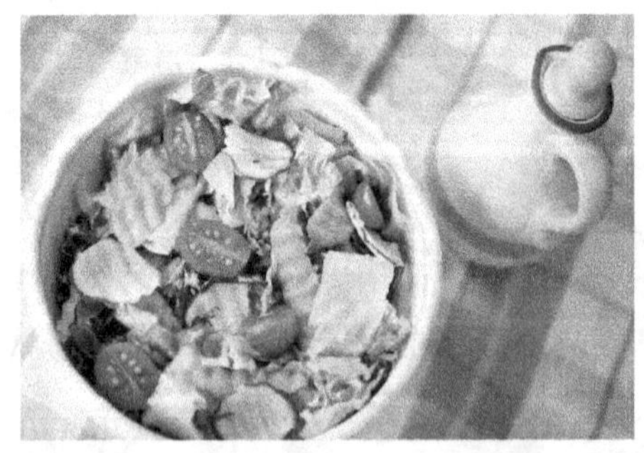

Recipe Adaptations And Substitutions

Recipe adaptations and substitutions are essential when following a vegan diet to replace animal-based ingredients with plant-based alternatives. Here are some common adaptations and substitutions for a vegan diet:

1. Dairy Substitutions:
- Milk: Replace cow's milk with plant-based milks like almond milk, soy milk, oat milk, or coconut milk.
- Butter: Use vegan margarine or plant-based butter substitutes.
- Cheese: Opt for vegan cheese alternatives made from nuts, soy, or tapioca starch.

2. Egg Substitutes:

- For binding: Use mashed bananas, applesauce, flaxseed meal, or chia seeds mixed with water as egg replacements.
- For leavening: Use baking powder or baking soda combined with vinegar or lemon juice.
- For structure: Silken tofu or vegan yogurt can provide structure in baked goods.

3. Meat Substitutes:

- Protein sources: Incorporate plant-based proteins such as tofu, tempeh, seitan, lentils, beans, chickpeas, or textured vegetable protein (TVP) in place of meat.
- Meat alternatives: Explore commercially available vegan meat alternatives like veggie burgers, vegan sausages, or plant-based "chicken" or "beef" substitutes.

4. Honey Substitutions:

- Use sweeteners like maple syrup, agave nectar, date syrup, or coconut nectar as replacements for honey.

5. Gelatin Substitutions:

-    Agar-agar, a seaweed-based gelatin substitute, can be used in place of traditional gelatin in recipes.

6. Fish Sauce Substitutions:

- Soy sauce, tamari, or liquid aminos can provide a savory and umami flavor in place of fish sauce.

7. Cream Substitutions:

- Coconut cream or cashew cream can be used as substitutes for heavy cream in recipes.

8. Yogurt Substitutions:

- Use dairy-free yogurt made from almond milk, soy milk, coconut milk, or cashews as a replacement for regular yogurt.

9. Worcestershire Sauce Substitutions:

- Vegan Worcestershire sauce or tamari sauce mixed with a bit of vinegar can be used as a substitute.

10. Recipe Adaptations:

- Modify recipes by replacing animal-based ingredients with plant-based alternatives, such as using vegetable broth instead of chicken broth or tofu or tempeh in place of meat in stir-fries or curries.

"Remember to check ingredient labels and choose vegan-certified products to ensure they are free from any animal-derived ingredients. With these adaptations and substitutions, you can create delicious and satisfying vegan versions of your favorite recipes"

CHAPTER 5

Embracing A Vegan Lifestyle

Embracing a vegan lifestyle refers to adopting a way of living that aligns with the principles and values of veganism. It involves making conscious choices to avoid the use of animal products, both in diet and other aspects of life, and instead, opting for plant-based alternatives.

At its core, embracing a vegan lifestyle goes beyond dietary choices and extends to ethical, environmental, and health considerations. Here are key aspects involved in embracing a vegan lifestyle:

1. Plant-Based Diet: A significant aspect of veganism is adopting a plant-based diet, which excludes all animal products such as meat,

poultry, fish, dairy, eggs, and honey. Instead, it emphasizes consuming fruits, vegetables, whole grains, legumes, nuts, and seeds as the primary sources of nutrition.

2. Ethical Considerations: Vegans often embrace the lifestyle due to ethical concerns for animals. They believe in respecting and avoiding the exploitation of animals for food, clothing, entertainment, or any other purposes. This includes avoiding products tested on animals and opting for cruelty-free alternatives.

3. Environmental Consciousness: Embracing a vegan lifestyle also stems from recognizing the environmental impact of animal agriculture. Animal farming contributes to deforestation, greenhouse gas emissions, water pollution, and habitat destruction. By choosing plant-based foods, vegans aim to reduce their carbon footprint and promote sustainable practices.

4. Health and Wellness: Many individuals adopt a vegan lifestyle for its potential health benefits. Vegan diets, when well-planned, can provide essential nutrients, fiber, and antioxidants while reducing the risk of certain chronic diseases like heart disease, diabetes, and certain cancers. It involves prioritizing whole, minimally processed foods and paying attention to proper nutrient balance.

5. Compassion and Advocacy: Embracing a vegan lifestyle often involves advocating for animal rights and promoting awareness about the benefits of veganism. Many vegans engage in community activities, educate others, and support organizations that align with their values.

6. Lifestyle Choices: Embracing a vegan lifestyle extends beyond food choices. It includes opting for cruelty-free and vegan products, such as cosmetics, clothing, and household items. Vegans strive to ensure that

their lifestyle aligns with their ethical beliefs and extends to all aspects of their lives.

It's important to note that embracing a vegan lifestyle is a personal choice, and individuals may have varying levels of commitment and approaches to veganism. Some may transition gradually, while others may adopt the lifestyle more swiftly. Ultimately, embracing a vegan lifestyle reflects a commitment to kindness, compassion, and making choices that align with one's values and respect for all living beings.

CONCLUSION

"The Ultimate Vegan Cookbook" serves as a valuable resource for individuals seeking to embrace a plant-based lifestyle or incorporate more vegan options into their diet. Throughout this cookbook, you will discover a diverse collection of delicious and nutritious recipes that showcase the incredible variety and flavors available in vegan cuisine.

By exploring the recipes and techniques provided, you can experience the benefits of a vegan diet, such as improved health, reduced environmental impact, and a compassionate approach to food choices. Whether you are a seasoned vegan, a curious beginner, or simply looking to add more plant-based meals to your repertoire, "The Ultimate Vegan Cookbook" offers a wealth of inspiration and practical guidance.

From energizing smoothie bowls to comforting soups, satisfying main dishes to delectable desserts, each recipe is thoughtfully crafted with plant-based ingredients to showcase the incredible culinary possibilities of vegan cooking. Moreover, the book provides valuable insights into vegan pantry essentials, recipe adaptations, and helpful tips for transitioning to a vegan lifestyle.

By embracing "The Ultimate Vegan Cookbook," you are embarking on a journey of creativity, nourishment, and mindful living. Every recipe not only nourishes your body but also respects the planet and its inhabitants. With each meal you prepare, you are contributing to a more sustainable, compassionate, and health-conscious way of eating.

So, let "This Cookbook" be your guide as you embark on this exciting culinary adventure. May it inspire you to explore new flavors, experiment with innovative ingredients, and discover the joy of creating wholesome, plant-based meals that are both satisfying and delicious. Enjoy the journey towards a vibrant, compassionate, and flavorful vegan lifestyle.

* 9 7 9 8 8 5 1 6 2 8 5 2 8 *